The Inheritance of Lactose Intolerance

By: Marsha Gujurati

~~~

Smashwords Edition

Prologue

The symptoms came on gradually. They began early in my 30s. I had occasional but severe heartburn. Once in a while, stomach cramps doubled me over. As I began the countdown to menopause, heartburn became weekly episodes. The doctor's test for gall bladder problems, based on the rising frequency of gut pain, proved nothing. The incidences of pain grew worse during peri-menopause.

I dismissed the pain as "something I ate," and let it go. As I've since learned, that was truer than I realized. It just wasn't the multiple foods I thought causing it all.

It was a chance comment from my 35-year-old manager that clued me in.

In a small, family-owned bead store, the day's shift was all women. While we bagged and tagged merchandise, we talked about food. The things we liked to cook, our favorite recipes, and what we had to avoid.

"I can't eat dairy products," the manager said. "Sometimes the cramps in my gut and chest hurt so bad that I think I'm going to die." She shook her head. "It always happens if I eat too much dairy."

"Like you're having a heart attack?" I asked. "Pain so bad that you're doubled over? Like I was the other day?" (I was at work when that happened.)

"Just like that," she said. "I can get away with a few mouthfuls once in a great while. But, not every day – and definitely not flat out milk stuff." She tilted her head. "You might want to look into it."

"But, I've always been able to drink milk."

"Humans aren't supposed to, though," she said.

"*What?*"

"Look it up," she said.

I blinked. "I wonder…"

What is Lactose Intolerance (LI)?

Lactose is a "double" sugar (disaccharide) in milk and milk products. An enzyme called lactase breaks down the lactose in the small intestine. You then have the two monosaccharides: glucose and galactose. From there, your body uses those sugars.

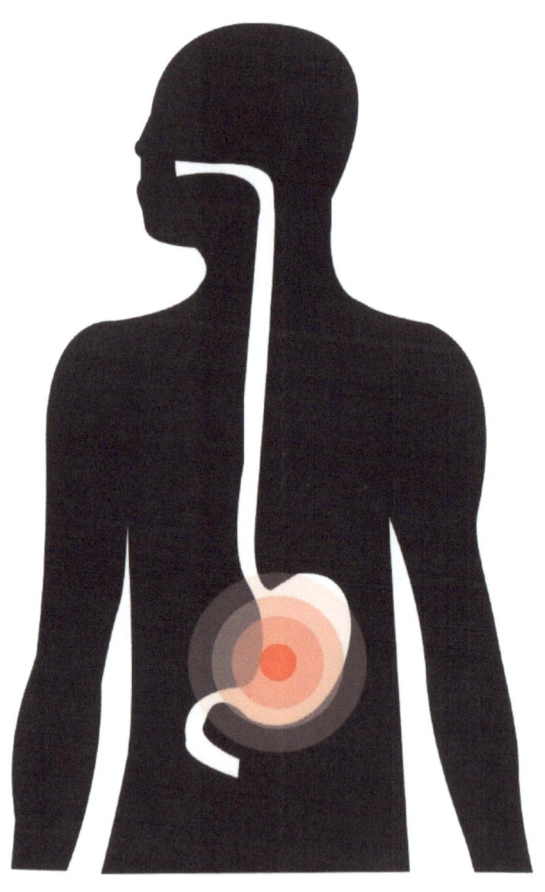

In *theory*, your body breaks down lactose. The *reality* – for most of us – is an inability to digest lactose. Instead of two monosaccharides, lactose sits in the gut and ferments. That, in turn, gives us a feeling of a bloated stomach which leads to passing excess gas. Or worse, it creates excruciating pain, cramps, and diarrhea. Nausea often follows on the heels of such gas or pain.

Many use the words "lactose intolerance" and "milk allergy" interchangeably. This is a disservice to those with a true food allergy. Granted, it's an easy out for those who don't want to explain their intolerance; it's still incorrect.

A true allergy (food or otherwise) engages the immune system. If not treated right away, you can go into anaphylactic shock which can kill you. Even if you do treat it immediately, some allergies are so severe (think bee stings or peanuts), that you'll die anyway.

Intolerance, however, involves some other part of your body. Milk, for instance, is a gastrointestinal problem. The immune system isn't on alert here. But, the small intestine sure is!

Most are angry when they find they can't eat dairy products anymore. They're also shocked at how many commercially prepared foods have dairy (of some sort) in them!

The scientific community has a new name for LI, one that puts a more precise spin on it: *lactase persistence*. It means that lactase, the enzyme that is *supposed* to decrease as we get older, doesn't. According to recent (and not-so-recent) studies, humans are the only species to drink milk as an adult. As science has learned, *we're not supposed to*. So, as long as we can tolerate lactose, we're still creating the enzyme. Otherwise, we're not.

What are the symptoms of LI?

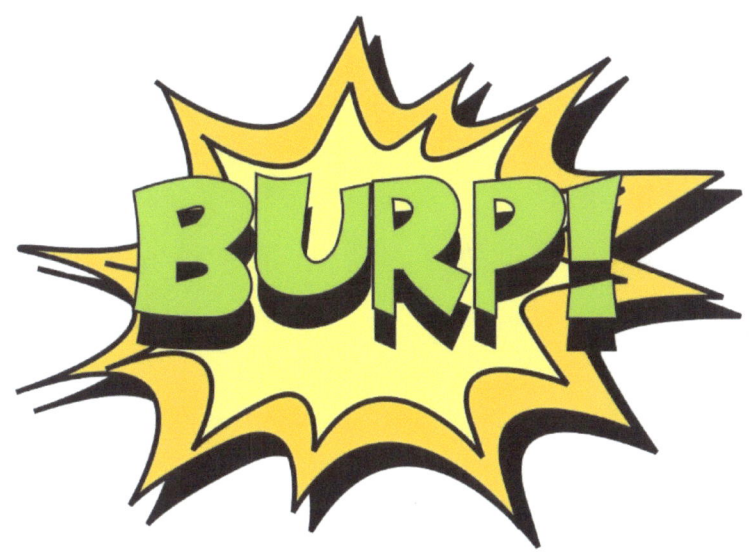

As mentioned above, look for these symptoms:

- Pain in the lower abdomen (lower intestine)
- Diarrhea
- Bloated stomach
- Extra gas
- Nausea
- Extreme heartburn

Some people have only one of them when they consume dairy, some have all of them, but most have only a few of them. The gut pain, the most common symptom, is excruciating. It effectively prevents people from going about their everyday lives until the symptoms pass, which takes anywhere between 6 and 10 hours later. Diarrhea, another common symptom, continues as long as you have too much dairy in your body.

How to learn if you have it or not

As with any disorder, a range of symptoms exist. Many mimic other disorders, including irritable bowel syndrome (IBS) and celiac disease. If you want to know for sure if you have LI, go to the doctor. He'll give you one of two tests. Both involve a lactose-laced drink (which will likely cause pain and/or gas if you are indeed LI), and a few hours:

- A breath test: how much hydrogen you have in your breath
- A blood test: how little sugar you have in your blood

If you do decide to go to the doctor, treat it as you would any other doctor's appointment. Bring lists:

- The medications you're taking, including any over-the-counter ones that you take regularly (Are you on an aspirin regime? Do you take vitamins?)
- Write down your symptoms, when they most often occur, how severe they are, and anything else that seems out of the ordinary
- Questions about your symptoms, about whether they could be something else, about the tests you might need to take

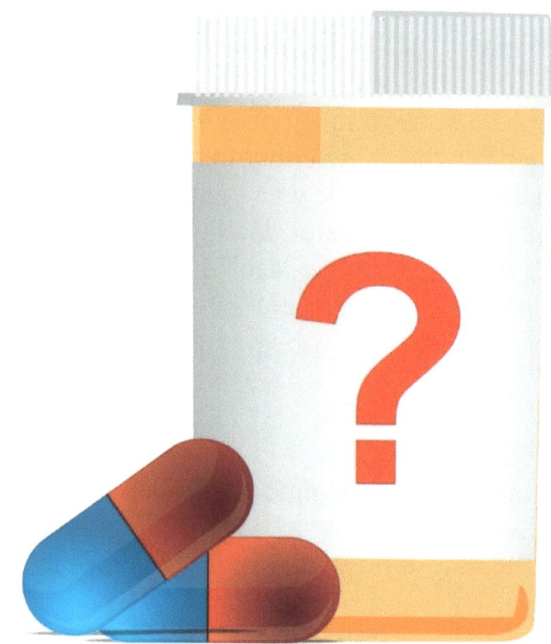

There is, of course, the old trial-and-error. It is *not* infallible. Doctors and the dairy industry both caution against such self-diagnosis, in case you have something more serious than LI. Nonetheless, if you want to try it this way, neither of them can actually stop you.

As I'm not a doctor, I'm passing along these links for your benefit. The first is a quiz put out by the Lady's Home Journal, the second by Medicine Net.

Lady's Home Journal:
http://www.lhj.com/lhj/quiz.jsp?quizId=/templatedata/lhj/quiz/data/LactoseIntolerance_Quiz_09082003.xml&catref=cat2810002&_requestid=273353

Medicine Net:
http://www.medicinenet.com/lactose_intolerance/page3.htm

What brings it on?

Most of the time, it's because of simply being human. It's mostly an inherited trait. The older we get, the more likely we are to develop it. Some, mostly premature babies, are born without much – or any – lactase, although even then it's rare. By the time a child enters school, lactase production has slowed. (There is some dispute as to the age that the intolerance begins; somewhere between age 3 and 13.) The best estimates show that roughly 2/3 (65%) of the human race are lactose intolerant.

According to the Mayo Clinic http://www.mayoclinic.org/diseases-conditions/lactose-intolerance/basics/definition/con-20027906, there are three types of lactose intolerance.

The first is a normal result of aging, as mentioned above. This is primary lactose intolerance. As you add different kinds of food to your diet, and you rely less on dairy, your lactase enzyme decreases.

The second can be the result of illness or injury, also known as secondary lactose intolerance. Infections of the lower intestine aggravate an already inherent situation. Bacteria, viruses, or parasites can create the "right" environment to make a person's lactase enzyme production shut down. Some of the diseases that "help" LI along are already diseases of the intestines, such as Crohn's disease, celiac disease, and gastroenteritis.

With congenital lactose intolerance (the third type), babies are born with a complete absence of lactase. Unfortunately, this disorder – called autosomal recessive inheritance – is passed down from generation to generation. The somewhat good news about this is that it takes both the mother and the father with the gene to pass it on.

Once you are lactose intolerant – whether by genetics, infection, or even age – you can't go back to being able to eat or drink as much dairy as you once did.

Is it curable?
Can lactose intolerant people ever eat dairy again?

Unfortunately, no drug or treatment is available to make your system create more lactase. The only reasonable relief is to refrain from eating dairy products. For some people, this will mean a permanent ban of all dairy. Most, however, can tolerate a few lactose-reduced products.

As mentioned above, many who are lactose intolerant can usually eat *some* dairy products. Not in huge quantities, but a little at a time. Except in those whose bodies can't absorb *any* lactose, many can eat the following *in small quantities* without ill effect:

- Hard cheeses (cheddar, parmesan), but not soft/"fresh" cheeses (mozzarella)
- Yogurt
- Sour cream
- Dairy products made with bacillus cultures

Why these? The lactose is already broken down in them. Your body can digest these more readily since there simply isn't much lactose in them.

This chart below explains some of the lactose and calcium in some foods (from WebMD

http://www.webmd.com/digestive-disorders/tc/lactose-intolerance-topic-overview)

	Approximate lactose and calcium in some foods[1]		
Food	**Serving size**	**Lactose (g)**	**Calcium (mg)**
Milk, fat-free	8 fl oz (240 mL)	12.5	300
Cheddar cheese	1 oz (30 g)	0.07	204
Cottage cheese, 2% milk fat	4 oz (113 g)	3	100
Cream cheese	1 oz (30 g)	0.9	28

Still, you don't want to get in the habit of eating too much too often. Lactose intolerance is in your body. Be aware of your eating habits in order to be as pain-free as possible.

Now, you can also include probiotics in your diet. These include the "live cultures" often found in yogurt. According to Clinical Trials (http://clinicaltrials.gov/show/NCT01593800), the main probiotics found in yogurt – the famed Lactobacillus acidophilus, Lactobacillus bulgaricus, and Streptococcus thermophilus – helped in the digestion of lactose. In another study, milk containing Bifidobacterium longum caused fewer problems than standard milk.

Logically speaking then, taking the pill form of probiotics will help as well. If, for example, you don't care for the tang of real yogurt (forget the flavored and sugared stuff), then it makes sense to take the probiotic in the more concentrated form of tablet or capsule.

What can you eat in a culture that consumes a lot of dairy?

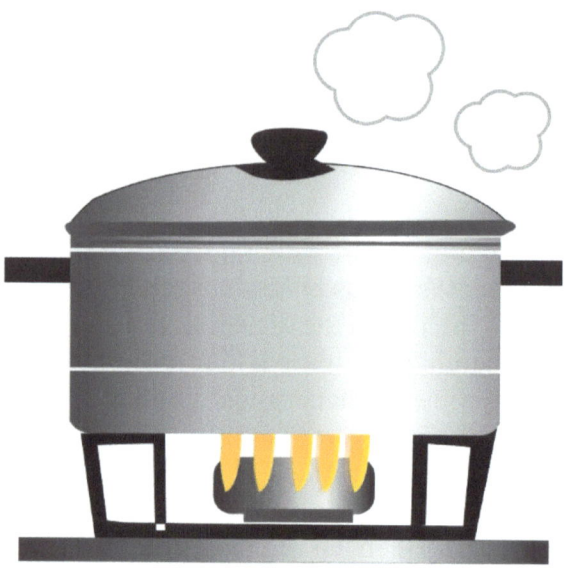

Dairy producers argue that dairy products are an absolute must for enough calcium. That isn't strictly true. Vegans make up 5% of Americans who don't drink or eat any kind of dairy. Many vegetarians don't either. They employ and enjoy plant-based calcium.

Foods that are high in calcium (and other valuable nutrients) include:

- Broccoli
- Pinto beans
- Spinach
- Rice milk
- Oranges

This is *not* an all-inclusive list of plant-based calcium. For that, I recommend studying the ways of vegans and vegetarians. Of course, it's a good idea to eat more vegetables anyway. These are simply a few of the best vegetables that supply of calcium. As I said, it isn't a complete list, so don't feel you must limit yourself to only these non-dairy foods for your calcium intake.

Here's a recipe for broccoli that uses sesame seeds (also high in calcium!):

In saucepan, combine

- 1 Tablespoon soy sauce
- 1 Tablespoon olive oil
- 1 Tablespoon apple cider vinegar
- 4 teaspoons sugar
- 1 Tablespoon toasted sesame seeds

Heat to boiling. Take it off the burner and pour it hot over a pound of fresh-steamed broccoli; turn spears to coat. Serve hot. Serves four.

What commercially prepared foods have dairy in them?

Nutrition Facts

Amount Per Serving

Calories 00   Calories from fat 0

	% Daily Value
Total Fat	0%
Saturated Fat 0g	0%
Trans Fat	0%
Cholesterol 0mg	
Sodium 0mg	
Total Carbohydrate 0mg	
Protein 0mg	

INGREDIENTS

Wheat flour Palm Oil Sugar Nibbed Almonds
Cornflour Baking Powder Skimmed Milk Salt
Glucose Syrup Flavoring Soya Leciti

Almost every week, watchdog groups contact the news with a story about a packaged, canned, or frozen food with hidden or potentially damaging ingredients (look no further than the dye industry!). One of the few that you don't hear about very often is dairy. Or its many permutations.

For example, "non-dairy" means it's less than 0.5% by weight. It doesn't mean "no dairy at all." Look at the ingredients on a canister of non-dairy coffee creamer. Its dairy product is sodium caseinate. Yes, that's a dairy product. It isn't enough to create hardship for most lactose intolerant people, but it can be quite the problem for those who are extremely sensitive and/or allergic to any milk products.

The following partial lists of lactose-containing foods are from the site: Food Allergy Research & Education (found at http://www.foodallergy.org/allergens/milk-allergy):

Some obvious places

- Milk (in all forms, including condensed, derivative, dry, evaporated, goat's milk and milk from other animals, low-fat, malted, milk fat, nonfat, powder, protein, skimmed, solids, whole, plus cream, buttermilk, and half-and-half)
- Butter, ghee, and buttermilk
- Cheese in all forms
- Sour cream, sour cream solids
- Yogurt

Some not-so obvious places

- Artificial butter flavor, and margarine
- Baked goods
- Chocolate
- Lactic acid starter culture and other bacterial cultures
- Non-dairy products

Some unexpected places where milk is sometimes found

- Some brands of canned tuna, and deli meats contain casein, a milk protein
- Many non-dairy products contain casein (a milk derivative), including non-dairy creamer
- Some specialty products made with milk substitutes (i.e., soy-, nut- or rice-based dairy products) are manufactured on equipment shared with milk
- Some medications contain milk protein

Again, these are just a few of the products on the market that have (or may have) some form of dairy in them. Look before you buy!

Is Lactose Intolerance on the rise?

According to several studies found online, Lactose Intolerance isn't so much on the rise as the fact that doctors have better methods of diagnosing disorders, diseases, allergies, intolerances, and so on.

Eli Roe (http://www.personal.psu.edu/afr3/blogs/siowfa13/2013/09/is-lactose-intolerance-on-the-rise.html) pointed out another possible explanation: an increase in immigration from countries with high rates of Lactose Intolerance.

Lactose Intolerance is historically connected by the consumption (or lack thereof) to cultural and ethnic groups. (See *Historically Speaking* further down for a more in-depth conversation.)

What products are available on the market to ease this intolerance?

Many people who are lactose intolerant don't want to give up dairy. For them, there are pills that you can simply swallow like any other pill. Chewable tablets exist as well; they are, however, as tasteful as chalk with the same texture. Be sure and follow the directions for using them.

Be aware, however, that these pills and chewables are stop-gap measures only. How effective they are depends entirely of your own lactase production or lack thereof. Sometimes, nothing works; that's a case of severe Lactose Intolerance. In a couple forums, people mentioned they sometimes increased the dosage on the labels in keeping with how much dairy they know they're going to eat. (Not recommended to do. Instead, keep your dairy intake down to more tolerable levels for yourself.)

The best measure of not having a stomach "attack" is to simply not drink or eat dairy products. It may not be the most enjoyable thing to do, but it's the most logical.

What brands carry lactose-free products?

Name brands of just the milk, such as Lactaid and Darigold are on the shelves now. Many stores carry their own brands of lactose-free milk. Kroger, Wal-Mart, and others carry their own store-brands of lactose-reduced or lactose-free milk.

Lactaid and Breyer's also make lactose-free ice cream. A real treat on those hot days! However, stores often carry only one brand or the other. Or, they may carry the milk, but not the ice cream.

As a side note, the FDA apparently has no direct definition for lactose-free (which means there is no direct regulation for it). However, the FDA *has* stated that "lactose-free… should not contain any lactose and a lactose-reduced… a meaningful reduction." This link shows how one company explains its use of "lactose-free" when – by FDA's words – it should be calling its milk "lactose-reduced":

https://www.truthinadvertising.org/great-value-lactose-free-milk/

Is Lactose Intolerance actually normal?

Historically, yes. Through archaeology, and historical studies, Lactose Intolerance is the norm, rather than modern-day intolerance. It's a mutated gene that allows your body to continue to create lactase long after your body were supposed to quit making it.

Science tends to follow the wisdom of ages, rather than be in the forefront. Scientists ask questions even when they see the proof that it exists, whatever the "it" happens to be. According to a project begun in 2009, and involving archaeologists, chemists and geneticists, science has learned that lactase persistence has been around since at least 7,500 years ago. For the most part, northern Europeans have the best developed "mutant gene" that helps them digest dairy.

It takes humans centuries to develop immunity against something. Lactose intolerance is something nearly all humans are born with. The northern Europeans are thought to be the first to develop it after taking up cow herding and dairy farming.

Historically Speaking:
Who is most susceptible to it?

Babies born full term tend to have the most lactase so that they can digest their mother's milk easily. After that, about age three, our bodies start producing less lactase. The break in having enough lactase to digest lactose, and not enough, becomes noticeable in most teens (although it's often ignored or misdiagnosed). Lactose Intolerance falls into further distinctions, such as ethnicity and gender.

Adults are the most likely to "get" it. It can begin with an infection in the lower intestine (bacterial or viral). It can also be from parasites (an animal living off us). It can begin as young as 3 or wait until you age, whether you're in your thirties, fifties, seventies or anything in between.

Any and all ethnicities are prone to it. According to studies in the 1970s, and backed up further by studies in the 2000s (past and ongoing), Caucasians are likely to get it after they're in school. Africans, Asians, Native Americans, Latinos – before school age.

The exact percentages of which culture / ethnicity suffer Lactose Intolerance more or less than another are not exact. They depend on various studies, which can vary in how they're conducted. Despite that, the different cultures are at relatively the same levels throughout the ongoing studies.

One of the more astounding things is that only 60% to 75% of the entire world is lactose intolerant. The reasoning is that, as ancestral northern Europeans depended more on dairy to survive, their genes mutated to accept the new food. Other cultures simply have not developed that gene because their diets didn't include a lot of dairy.

How much lactose can a culture / ethnic group actually tolerate? This much:

- 0% to 5% = Native American and Asian peoples
- 25% = African and Caribbean peoples
- 50% = Mediterranean peoples
- 90% = Northern European (which means most American Caucasians) peoples

According to one report, Sweden's percentage of those who can drink dairy is one of the highest. (http://abcnews.go.com/Health/WellnessNews/story?id=84 50036)

See also this link (http://www.nature.com/polopoly_fs/1.13471!/menu/main/t opColumns/topLeftColumn/pdf/500020a.pdf (PDF)) about how prevalent dairy was to the northern Europeans. An archaeology team of researchers included a paleogeneticist, a bioarchaeologist, a geochemist, as well as the original archaeologist who began to study his finds.

One of the finds concluded that since the Mediterraneans started using dairy thousands of years ahead of Europeans, those ancient people found a way to reduce the lactose in milk. Most likely it was fermentation into cheeses and yogurts.

Now, as an alternative, some people with cow's milk LI can digest *goat's* milk. The hypothesis behind this is that the lactose particles in goat's milk are smaller, and therefore more easily digested. It tends to leave behind less lactose in the intestines to ferment.

This article also suggests that one-in-ten people may be intolerant of a specific and major protein in cow's milk: alpha S1 casein protein. Goat's milk (and mother's milk) doesn't have it. (See this: http://www.dynamicchiropractic.com/mpacms/dc/article.php?id=38646)

Opposing Viewpoints

In two separate PDFs, the dairy industry suggests that lactose intolerance isn't as prevalent as lactose maldigestion, also known as primary lactase deficiency. They don't deny that LI exists. They simply take the point of view that the maldigestion is far more likely than LI, or even a true milk allergy. (One of the papers says that milk allergy may be outgrown.)

Many people use an elimination diet to discover whether they are or aren't lactose intolerant. They don't go to the doctor for a clinical diagnosis. As a result, the UK Dairy Council lays claim that these people are "using information based on unfounded preconceptions." Their next statement implies that only those 2% who go to their doctors for clinical diagnoses are real sufferers.

Both PDFs suggest that no one needs to eliminate all dairy products. Regardless what you call it, maldigestion or intolerance, all people can eat *some* form of dairy. Some can eat more, some less, but all can eat dairy in one form or another. "No one needs to be lactose intolerant."

They admitted that certain cultural groups (specifically Africans, Asians, and Native Americans) are more likely to have higher lactose maldigestion. At the same time, they insist that these cultures are able to learn to drink milk.

See these links for further information:

http://www.nationaldairycouncil.org/SiteCollectionDocume
nts/LI%20and%20Minorites_FINALIZED.pdf

http://www.efsa.europa.eu/en/efsajournal/doc/1777.pdf

Controversy Over rBST or rBHT How much of rBST or rBHT (cow hormone) contributes to LI?

The addition of rBHT or rBST (lab-created cow hormones) stands accused of creating LI. That the milk is "dirty" is one thing (more on that later). That it has anything in particular to do with lactose intolerance is incorrect. That misconception is because it appears that, since using additional hormones in milk, LI is on the rise. Since you are what you eat, it makes a certain kind of logic.

However, in this case, the raging hormones (both literal and debate), and LI aren't connected. As explained before, doctors are now better equipped to understand LI-type complaints, and have tests for them.

Based on the old-but-still-true adage, "We are what we eat," then anything added to your food will in turn get into us. That holds true for rBST and rBHT. The addition of hormones to cows (and the overuse of antibiotics to cure the diseases the hormones create) means more hormones in us. Our bodies try to use what we feed it. In other words, it doesn't help us to have it in us.

See these links:

http://www.allergykids.com/uncategorized/raging-hormones/
http://www.pearlsofnutrition.com/blog/category/nutrition
http://www.ejnet.org/bgh/nogood.html

However, of all the things rBST and rBHT have against them, creating LI or prolonging lactase persistence isn't among the reasons. Those hormones haven't anything to do with the breakdown of lactase production. As mentioned before, lactase is naturally supposed to cease after a certain age.

Forums and Blogs

While poking around on the internet, I found a few forums and blogs. Unfortunately, the forums were ill-attended. The blogs weren't up to date.

One forum had a recent (July 2014) remark. Before that, however, the remark was in January 2014, and before that, October 2013. The rest weren't any more attended, even those on medical sites.

Just as scant were the blogs. Many started, none current. Posts were months old; some looked completely abandoned.

Take a look around, however. You may find some good ones, some *current* forums and blogs that I missed.

Humor

There is, however, a light note to all this "doom and gloom" about lactose intolerance. As the old saying goes, "Laugh, and the world laughs with you."

http://www.buzzfeed.com/gabrielakruschewsky/lactose-intolerance-is-the-worst

http://www.buzzfeed.com/rachelysanders/dairy-free-treats

Disclaimer

Appendix

(a complete list of the links used in this book)

General

Mayo Clinic

http://www.mayoclinic.org/diseases-conditions/lactose-intolerance/basics/definition/con-20027906

ABC News

http://abcnews.go.com/Health/WellnessNews/story?id=8450036

WebMD

http://www.webmd.com/digestive-disorders/tc/lactose-intolerance-topic-overview

http://www.webmd.com/digestive-disorders/ss/slideshow-calcium (slideshow)

http://www.webmd.com/digestive-disorders/lactose-intolerance-directory (useful links in this directory)

National Library of Medicine

http://www.pcrm.org/health/diets/vegdiets/what-is-lactose-intolerance

http://www.ncbi.nlm.nih.gov/pubmedhealth/PMH0005145/

http://www.nlm.nih.gov/medlineplus/ency/article/000276.htm

Food Allergy Research & Education (FARE)

http://www.foodallergy.org/allergens/milk-allergy

Medicine Net

http://www.medicinenet.com/lactose_intolerance/page3.htm

Dynamic Chiropractic (article re goat's milk)

http://www.dynamicchiropractic.com/mpacms/dc/article.php?id=38646

13 Home Remedies

http://health.howstuffworks.com/wellness/natural-medicine/alternative/alternative-treatments-for-lactose-intolerance-ga1.htm

Food Health Innovation (PDF): (European Industry Position Paper)

http://www.foodhealthinnovation.com/media/8091/industry_position_paper_-_lactose_free.pdf

SiOWfa13

http://www.personal.psu.edu/afr3/blogs/siowfa13/2013/09/is-lactose-intolerance-on-the-rise.html

BBN

http://blackandbrownnews.com/lifestyle/what-is-lactose-intolerance-and-what-causes-it-take-a-quiz/

Lady's Home Journal (Quiz)

http://www.lhj.com/lhj/quiz.jsp?quizId=/templatedata/lhj/quiz/data/LactoseIntolerance_Quiz_09082003.xml&catref=cat2810002&_requestid=273353

FDA standards regarding 100% lactose-free

https://www.truthinadvertising.org/great-value-lactose-free-milk/

Historically Speaking

Nature

http://www.nature.com/news/archaeology-the-milk-revolution-1.13471

http://www.nature.com/news/2007/070226/full/news070226-4.html

http://www.nature.com/polopoly_fs/1.13471!/menu/main/topColumns/topLeftColumn/pdf/500020a.pdf (PDF)

Opposing Viewpoint

Dairy Reporter

http://www.dairyreporter.com/Markets/Dairy-authority-raises-doubts-over-lactose-intolerance-claims

National Dairy Council (PDF)

http://www.nationaldairycouncil.org/SiteCollectionDocuments/LI%20and%20Minorites_FINALIZED.pdf

European Food Safety Authority

http://www.efsa.europa.eu/en/efsajournal/doc/1777.pdf

Humor

Buzzfeed

http://www.buzzfeed.com/gabrielakruschewsky/lactose-intolerance-is-the-worst

http://www.buzzfeed.com/rachelysanders/dairy-free-treats

Controversy

Pearls of Nutrition

http://www.pearlsofnutrition.com/blog/category/nutrition

Allergy Kids

http://www.allergykids.com/uncategorized/raging-hormones/

Ejnet.org

http://www.ejnet.org/bgh/nogood.html

About the Author

Marsha Gujurati is an avid researcher of anything health or wellness related. She prefers to spend her time, cozied up with her laptop researching alternative therapies and medical practices.

Other books by this author

Please visit your favorite Ebook retailer to discover other books by Melissa Jones

It Comes Natural
The Best Foods for Your Sex Life
The Inheritance of Lactose Intolerance

And many more!

www.ingramcontent.com/pod-product-compliance
Lightning Source LLC
Chambersburg PA
CBHW050842290526
45792CB00001B/495